Aging in Place

Donna Christner-Lile

Aging in Place

Safely living in your
"Home Sweet Home" until you're 100+

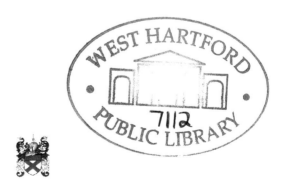

TATE PUBLISHING & *Enterprises*

The opinions expressed by the author are not necessarily those of Tate Publishing, LLC.

This book is designed to provide accurate and authoritative information with regard to the subject matter covered. This information is given with the understanding that neither the author nor Tate Publishing, LLC is engaged in rendering legal, professional advice. Since the details of your situation are fact dependent, you should additionally seek the services of a competent professional.

Published by Tate Publishing & Enterprises, LLC
127 E. Trade Center Terrace | Mustang, Oklahoma 73064 USA
1.888.361.9473 | www.tatepublishing.com

Tate Publishing is committed to excellence in the publishing industry. The company reflects the philosophy established by the founders, based on Psalm 68:11,
"The Lord gave the word and great was the company of those who published it."

Book design copyright © 2011 by Tate Publishing, LLC. All rights reserved.
Cover design by Blake Brasor
Interior design by Sarah Kirchen

Published in the United States of America

ISBN: 978-1-61777-603-8
Self-Help / Aging
11.06.07

I dedicate this book to my mother, Alta Christner. She has always been my best advocate. In no small way she taught me the concept of facing the challenges of life with her profound phraseology, "You can't learn to swim by standing on the bank." She has astounded others with her willingness to try new surroundings and ways of being in late life. It's a joy and privilege to be able to call her mother. With her Christian kindness and compassion, she is a laudable example of a wonderful mother.

> "Pray for those who are very old, for they have come a long way. Pray for those who are very young, for they have a long way to go. Pray for those in between, for they are doing the work."
>
> —*Nelson Mandela*

ACKNOWLEDGMENTS

No author could complete his or her work without the love of family, friends, and cohorts. My husband, Dennis, daily affirms me with love and encouragement, making it possible for me to move forward. When I feel least like presenting the world with this work or any other, he is always there to encourage and support me. My son, Brett, and daughter-in-law, Sabrina, have always had faith and encouragement for Mother, no matter what pathway I chose. Sally Gelardin, Ph.D., is one of the finest mentors a transitional counselor could ever have—always available and always encouraging. Thank you, Sherline Montgomery, for prayers, patience, and expertise in the edit. Mickey Morales and Becky Bartunek are two of my favorite fans. Without their love and support this book would have taken another year to finish. Of course, kudos to Jordan Sangalang, a young fourteen-year-old budding artist with his adorable interpretations of the illustrations I requested. I have not attempted to cite in the text all the authorities and sources consulted in the preparation of this manual. To do so would require more space than is available. The list would include departments of various governments, libraries, industrial institutions, periodicals, and many individuals.

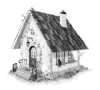

TABLE OF
CONTENTS

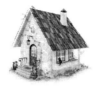

FOREWORD

By: Sally Gelardin, Ed.D.

A decade ago I co-presented with my husband at a workshop on senior co-housing. A year ago, I was interviewed on the topic of "Caregiving and Career." However, it was not until this year that the plight of seniors' living situations hit home.

Having recently helped move my ninety-nine-year-old father-in-law and his ninety-eight-year-old wife from a home in Washington to an assisted-living facility in Arizona, I am experiencing firsthand the dilemmas that author Donna Christner-Lile addresses. As she speaks of elders falling being the primary motivator for moving from their homes, I reflect on an incident with my father-in-law. In the middle of the night, he attempted to get up to go to the bathroom and lost his balance because he was so weak. I managed to help him back onto the couch (where he was sleeping) but could not move the heavy furniture closer to the couch to prevent another fall. Instead, I spent the rest of the night sitting up at the base of the couch, ready to catch him if he fell again (not a very good solution for a one-hundred-and-ten-pound woman with small bones). Then I visited him at the assisted-living facility. He fell again. This time I could not help him up, because he was dead weight—he did not have any strength left. Fortunately, he had a good sense of humor both times. Now, an artillery of caregivers has been arranged to assist the elderly couple. We learn as we go.

In a couple days, I shall join my eighty-seven-year-old mother, who is visiting my two brothers and their retired wives, in Florida. During the visit, we shall visit retirement homes and assisted-living facilities. Mom has lived in western Massachusetts her entire life; but her friends are getting older, and both she and her friends are becoming less mobile. For the first time she is considering moving near her sons, one of which is a doctor. She would not even consider moving near me in California because she knows I am still working in high gear.

As I approach the sixth decade of my life, I contemplate my later years—where, how, and with whom I shall live? Ms. Christner-Lile notes that aging is easier if one can stay in one's home if the home is adapted to elderly needs and if one is surrounded by family, friends, and excellent service providers. In addition, aging in place, to me, means carrying one's home in one's heart or adapting to life changes with grace—not always an easy task, even with all the sources of support suggested by the author.

Ms. Christner-Lile provides a valuable resource for both family caregivers and for those of us who are approaching our later years. She has both the personal and professional experience to write about aging in place. With a background in both real estate and life transition counseling, she has expertise to talk about both environmental and emotional issues that can arise during the aging process. Although she describes me as her mentor, I consider us co-mentors. I learn from her as much, or more, than she has ever learned from me. This little gem of a book is packed with priceless tips for both aging adults and their caregivers.

Dr. Sally Gelardin owns Aging Works, a consulting organization for baby boomers on up who are experiencing career and life transitions. She is an international speaker on lifework-balancing issues, provider of several career certification and CEU training programs, women's studies portfolio evaluator at the University of San Francisco, and author of two books: *The Mother-Daughter Relationship: Activities for Promoting Life work Success* (CAPS press, 2004) and *Starting and Growing a Business in the New Economy: Successful Career Entrepreneurs Share Stories and Strategies.* (National Career Development Association, 2007). Websites: www.lifeworkps.com/sallyg, www.jobjuggler.net, www.AskDrSal.com

INTRODUCTION

Increasingly, boomers, elders, and caregivers are expressing concerns about, and have questions related to, the best living arrangements for later life. This book is meant to be a simple yet comprehensive guide that you can use to help you preplan to live in your home forever. I hope it inspires action on your part rather than a feeling of being overwhelmed. Sometimes opening a conversation about where and how aging parents will live in later years is as uncomfortable for adult children as the parent/child "sex talk" at puberty was for parents. This book can work as a catalyst to open conversations about the subjects that you find difficult to discuss with your loved ones. In this guide you will find answers to your questions and lists of resources and worksheets to meet your needs. I have a very no-nonsense approach to this subject. It is my heartfelt desire that this book will make conversations with your children or parents about aging in place easier and imminent.

THE REALITY OF AGING IN PLACE

In 1998, John Weicher, a senior research fellow at Hudson Institute, indicated that America's elderly wanted to continue living in their own homes and neighborhoods. However, in 2006, the retiring boomer's preference was to live independently yet increasingly close to grandchildren. "Moving closer to grown children and grandchildren is a new option for retirees,[1]" says Elinor Ginzler, manager for independent living and long-term care for AARP. AARP does not keep official statistics on this category, but Ms. Ginzler says that she can see it happening all over the country. Families are choosing to relocate to be near one another after no longer needing to live in the vicinity of previously held jobs.[2] Unfortunately the boomer retirees are moving to be close to their children, not the parents. These adult children have often moved frequently in their careers, and thus moving isn't a traumatic event to them. Boomers feeling of "home" is where their children are. This change in family dynamic is quite different from the days of the Walton's, when there were so many on the farm, and stayed on the farm, that someone was always available to help the parents. Many older adults, 80+ resist moving, feeling they will be leaving their lifelong friends; however, often the lifelong friends are aging too, with needs of their own; those friends cannot always be there when their friend needs support.

Our society has wonderful highways and street systems. However, with the volume of traffic using the roads, another toll is taken in stress when adult children are trying to "be there" for all the aging parent's necessary needs. I know adult children who travel many hours every day to commute to work stop by to be sure their aging parent checked their blood sugar and ate properly, yet they had to hurry to pick up their own children from school. Boomers and their children live in a very fast-paced and stressful society. We taught them to be responsible to their family. We taught them to be good employees so they could make a living to take care of themselves. In order for them to be effective spouses and parents as well as earn enough money to pay for their own retirement, we owe it to them to pre-plan to be safe and independent as we age. In most situations it is asking too much for our children to be *daily* caregivers, given today's demands to meet their responsibilities.

Another trend I see is that of boomer retirees who are anxious to move out of their homes in metro areas to less expensive areas. Unfortunately, many were so caught up with the excitement of the low prices in the new area that they didn't do their homework. They were just thinking of that dream home they could build. For many, soon after moving into their dream home, they needed knee replacements, back surgery, etc. Often they didn't buy the new home with the thought of possible declining physical capabilities. They may not have considered impaired mobility accessibility in their dream home design. Often the quieter rural areas lack the availability of local services needed to be independent in late life. Thus, many had to change their plans and move close to their children. The dream home had to be sold because it wasn't age-in-place ready, and they had not done their homework prior to moving. Pre-planning is everything!

It is important to state that aging in place will not be an option for all people, because of cognitive decline or lack of support; however, education on preplanning your retirement household to age in place will increase the chances of you being able to do so.

For example, according to numerous studies, falls are the major reason for hospitalization among the elderly.[3][4] After a fall, or for other medical reasons, a hospital stay is likely in the future for many elders. After hospitalization, many never return home. The typical progression is to a rehab facility, then to a nursing home because their own homes no longer meet their needs. The factor of accessibility for impaired mobility mentioned earlier is very important. Having the knowledge provided in this book will help you start making arrangements so that your home and support staff will be ready if necessary. If you are a Boomer moving to be closer to grandchildren or if you are an older adult and want to stay in your current home, wouldn't you rather go home after a hospital stay than to a skilled nursing facility?

All of the following suggestions are most beneficial if addressed *before* housing decisions are made. Unless you are independently wealthy, making decisions after moving or remodeling can be costly and often limit your financial ability to age where you desire. This is not the time in your life to be impulsive! Making needed structural changes, finding outside support options, and finding funds to pay for support *after* an unexpected hospitalization are too overwhelming because it's too late! Here are suggestions to start a realistic consideration of aging in place. Take the proactive approach of preplanning in order to break the pattern of hospital, to rehab, to skilled nursing facility. Plan forward with confidence knowing you can go home to recuperate after any disability or fall. Consider the four primary factors: health, support, safety, and finances.

NOTES

_____

_____

_____

_____

_____

_____

_____

_____

_____

_____

_____

_____

_____

_____

_____

_____

_____

_____

CONSULT WITH YOUR DOCTOR

In making all decisions for major changes in lifestyle, your primary physician should be consulted first. Often physicians and other professional health providers, who provide primary care to the elderly, are the first professionals to become aware of a problematic home situation, either through their own observations or by report from a concerned family member. They have become experts in the most common problems. With preventative planning, it's only reasonable to consult with them on your journey to age in place. The doctor will give you an assessment of your present medical conditions, taking into consideration your familial genetic history. After consultation with the doctor, construct a plan for your home environment to adequately prevent accidents and facilitate care. You are designing your home environment to accommodate the most likely disabilities *you* might encounter that would prevent *you* from staying in your home.

On the next page you will find a helpful worksheet to take with you to the doctor's office on your next appointment. If you have more than one physician, it is wise to allow all of them to give you input on the worksheet.

Medical Evaluation Worksheet

QUESTIONS TO CONSIDER WITH YOUR DOCTOR	COMMENTS
1. What is your current physical condition? Excellent, Good, Fair, Poor	
2. Do you have conditions/signs that suggest future impairment?	
3. What are the impairments related to your familial genetic history?	
4. Are you aware of the possible side effects (such as poor coordination or lack of balance) of the medications you are taking?	
5. Do you need a bone density test? Ask about medications that can strengthen your bones and make them less likely to break.	
6. Are there any other tests he/she suggests?	
7. Are you currently in an exercise program?	
8. Have you had a vision test lately? If so, did you take care of any impaired vision?	
9. Are there modifications to your home that you should make in advance to prepare for your future health?	

NOTES

CHECK YOUR SUPPORT SYSTEM

Family

It is estimated that family and friends are the sole source of physical assistance for nearly three-quarters of impaired older adults in a community. That's seventy-five percent! Family and friends are also the elder's preferred source of non-financial help.[5] The services that family caregivers provide for "free" are estimated to be $257 billion a year. That is twice as much as is actually spent on homecare and nursing home services combined.[6]

One current trend, cited by Harris Interactive, suggests that "grand boomers" (boomers with grandchildren) are choosing to age in place (independently) because they desire to stay near family and friends.[7] [8] Because of increased longevity and better health, these grandparents are active, involved, and resolute in relating to their grandchildren. Grand boomers now have an influence over their grandchildren and great-grandchildren longer than any generation of grandparents that came before them. [9]

One should give realistic and considerable thought to the caregiver's (family member's) availability. In the past, there have been studies alluding to the fact that caregivers can incur significant loss in career development, salary, retirement income, and substantial out-of-pocket expenses as a result of caregiving. A Rice University study indicated that women who assume caregiving responsibilities face serious economic consequences: loss of salary and benefits due to quitting a job, loss of pay from reducing hours on the job or working part time, loss of promotion opportunities that require more hours on the job, and loss of training opportunities that require travel, just to name a few. Their study showed that middle-aged women (aged fifty-one to sixty-one years) who assumed caregiving roles for their aging parents were two and a half times more likely than non-caregivers to end up living in poverty; they were five times more likely to receive public assistance through SSI when they were older themselves.

Single women had an even higher risk. They were four times more likely than marked caregivers to live in poverty in later life. Women are less likely to be able to afford to leave the work force due to need for income, yet they are typically the ones who do leave to care for family.[10] So when we are considering family as caregivers, we must realistically consider their future in this plan.

Dr. Dale Atkins brilliantly states in her book, *I'm OK, You're My Parents*:

> A lot of times parents are making decisions out of their own needs. They want to be in the vicinity of their grandchildren. They want to know as they get older and natural aging occurs, they will be closer to their children. Those are realistic ideas in their own minds, but they may not have discussed it with their children.

Meanwhile, the adult children may have expectations of their own. Ms. Atkins says, "One might think about a built-in baby sitter and forget old feuds or that the parents never liked her husband." [11] Ah, yes! If a caregiver and his/her loved one *avoid discussing this issue together, then they are planning for failure!* This topic is like having an elephant in the room.

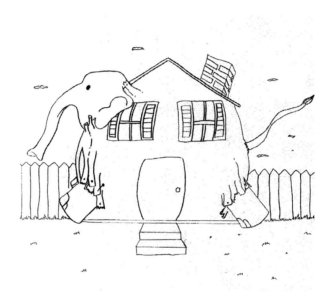

Addressing the quality of life for the caregiver is very important, because if the caregiver reaches burnout, there will be no advocate for the elder. This elephant grows on pretense of well-being and lack of honest communication. This elephant will destroy the tranquility of the household and deplete the well-being of what could have been a very good caregiver for a senior.

This is truly not a time in our nation's history for elders to be alone in advocating for their medical and daily needs. (Anyone who has navigated the enigmatic computer system for Medicare Prescription Drugs can tell you that!)

AARP brings up another good point—if you are thinking of moving close to your children: "Moving to a community with social opportunities and support puts you in a situation where you are not 100 percent dependent on your kids. We need to give consideration to whether we would be happy living where the children are, even if the children move away or if moving again is an option." So if your adult children are still in their career promotion years, you need to discuss that question with them. Don't make the mistake of assuming you are putting your children first by not asking them to help. I don't know of a family member who doesn't want the privilege of helping his family, yet every circumstance is different. Give the children the option of telling you what they can handle. On the other hand, should you mistakenly take the attitude that "you raised them, and now it's their turn to take care of you," it could be problematic for them and you. Burnout or guilt is a prescription for unhappiness.

One option is to call in a mentor. Counselors trained in life transitions specialize in the development of adults through each life stage. You want one specializing in mid-to-late life. Typically, they are certified by the National Board for Certified Counselors (NBCC). You can find them by going to the website www.nbcc.org. They are experts at helping families reflect realistically and honestly to what roles each member will be playing. With defined roles, the possibility of misunderstandings or problems will be minimized. For my clients I design a life-care plan so they know who will take care of them and how they will finance it throughout their life continuum.

Get the elephant out of the room early!

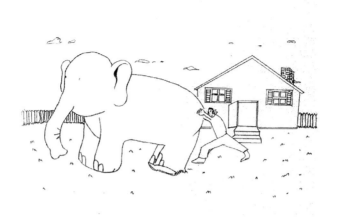

On the following pages are tips suggested for your caregiver to balance work, family, and caregiving recommended by the US Department of Health and Human Services.

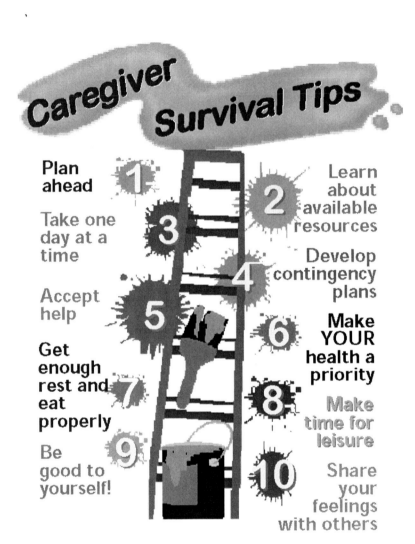

Caregiver Survival Tips

1. Plan ahead
2. Learn about available resources
3. Take one day at a time
4. Develop contingency plans
5. Accept help
6. Make YOUR health a priority
7. Get enough rest and eat properly
8. Make time for leisure
9. Be good to yourself!
10. Share your feelings with others

Resources

AoA's National Eldercare Locator: 1–800–677–1116

www.eldercare.gov

Your local area agency on aging: Eldercare
Locator or your local telephone directory

Family Caregiver Alliance: www.caregiver.org

National Alliance for Caregiving:
www.caregiving.org

Alzheimer's Association: www.alz.org

National Family Caregivers Assn:
www.nfcacares.org

AARP:www.aarp.org
Phone: (202) 619–0724
Fax: (202) 260–1012
E-mail: aoainfo@aoa.gov

U.S. Department of Health and Human Services

Friends

Neighbors and friends are usually willing to help. However, their limitations could impede the twenty-four-seven care you might possibly need. Again, honestly discussing with your friends how they might feel about helping you with grocery shopping, doctors' appointments, social events, etc., is imperative. Keep in mind how reliable they are; neither you nor your caregiver can constantly be looking for alternative sources of help if someone doesn't show up. Sensitivity to the honest answers your friends give you is key. Possibly using the trained mentor would be best. You are welcome to contact me at 2mentor@mentorcentral.com if you cannot find a qualified counselor.

Alternative Services

Almost every city in America today has a system of human services for seniors. Often in rural communities they are provided by a larger neighboring community. These programs are designed to help seniors stay independent and socialized. Become familiar with the services available in *your* community before you make decisions to live there. Those who work in senior services know that isolation is an enemy of good senior health. They also know the services they provide can give much-needed time and rest to the caregivers of the individuals they serve.

Support System

QUESTION	YES	NO	CONTACT NAME, PHONE, COMMENTS
1. Do you have a friend who can assist you? Do they drive?			
2. Does your friend have impairments that would make it difficult to help you?			
3. What type of assistance do you need? Shopping, doctors apts., laundry, cooking, a.m. or p.m. grooming?			
4. If your friend is unable to assist you with these things, would you consider hiring outside help?			
5. Does the local city/county government have senior support services?			
6. Is there a senior center in the community?			
7. Does the community have a Meals on Wheels program?			
8. Is there a senior "para transit" system in the community?			
9. Is there a "ride along" program?			
10. Is there a bill paying service?			
11. Is there a grocery store that delivers?			
12. Does the pharmacy deliver?			

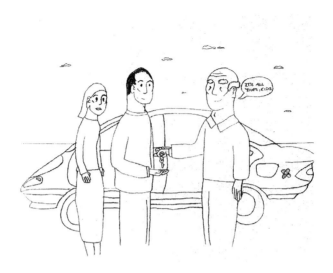

Are you seeing some new dings on the car or are your friends not accepting rides from you anymore? Are you occasionally getting confused on how to get home?

The services provided to the senior community are designed to keep the senior independent and socialized without the need for the caregiver to drive. Knowing where these systems are *before* moving into a community is important. Any local government will have the information you need to find this support. Following are some of the services that may be available in your community:

1. Many communities have paratransit systems to assist in getting the senior out to social activities, doctors' appointments, or anywhere they want to go. A paratransit is usually a van or bus. They are designed to accommodate anyone with or without wheelchairs or other mobility aids. The senior can set up his/her ride by phone and go to any destination he/she chooses. Paratransit drivers are alert to the needs of the elders and are able to assist them on and off the vehicle.

This gives the senior the independence he or she wants and lowers the stress level of the caregiver. The caregiver doesn't have to make arrangements to leave work or have to make a choice to be with the children at their activities or drive you somewhere. If independence is what you want, this is a good way to get it.

2. Some seniors have said the transit services seem slow; they have to wait longer than they would like. Given the choice of interrupting the caregiver at work or waiting a little longer—is a choice the senior must make.

3. Some communities have "ride-a-longs." Occasionally seniors need assistance on their journeys. A"Ride-a-long" is a volunteer from the community who accompanies paratransit riders to the store or doctor's office, wherever they want to go. Thus you have your independence and the caregiver has respite.

4. Senior support services are often in the form of Meals on Wheels. This is basic good nutrition—a full lunch and usually enough for dinner. When your caregiver can depend on you eating a very good lunch, plus knowing someone was there to visit and see how you are, the caregiver can be more relaxed. Senior support services ease the stress on your caregiver.

5. Friendly visitor programs are often included in senior services. Individuals are trained by human services to be interesting companions. Seniors who don't get out as much as they used to can have a friendly visitor stop by to visit. Many times they will go to lunch or movies, will play cards, or just visit. The caregiver knows his/her senior has company and doesn't feel guilty by not stopping by all the time. With the friendly visitor program for support, the senior achieves independence, and the caregiver achieves guilt-free respite.

6. Visiting nurses. One of the most exciting services I found recently was a program where nursing students were sent out every day to check the blood sugar of diabetes patients who were enrolled in the program. This gives reassurance to the family that someone was seeing their loved one and checking on their health needs.

7. Senior centers are available in most communities. Senior centers are great meeting areas that provide socialization and learning opportunities for seniors who want to get out and have some fun. My mother was always happy to be with people her own age for a while rather than be constantly in the world of fifty-somethings. She said it was so comforting to spend time with people who remembered the good old days personally, not from a history book.

8. Many cities have a bill paying service for individuals who can no longer keep up with monthly mail. These services hire bonded individuals to go to your home and assist on a monthly basis to keep the bill paying up-to-date. The caregiver no longer has to worry that their loved one might forget to pay a bill and have vital services disrupted. These organizations can be found from your local city Human Services Department. If your area doesn't have a Human Services Department, go to the phone book or Internet and call the local Council on Aging or the National Council on Aging (www.NCOA.org).

9. Most cities have access to AARP's Taxaide service. This service is comprised of nearly 32,000 IRS certified volunteers staffing 8,000 sites across the United States. They give tax preparation services to the seniors. Usually they can be found at senior centers. If not, find the nearest location at the AARP website: www.aarp.org/money/taxaide.

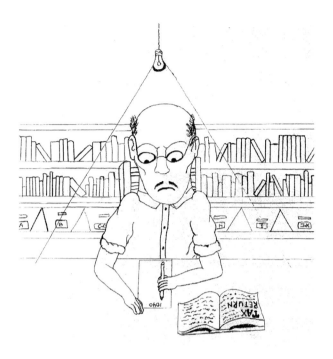

There are many more services available. If you call Human Services in your area, you will be directed to any and all at-home services that you might want from time to time. It would be listed as the City of [your city name] Human Services. In rural communities, the local fire station or sheriff's office has the information on senior services available in the area. Discharge planners and social workers at local hospitals often have this information too.

Obviously, this gives a high degree of independence and time to *enjoy* family and friends, rather than having loved ones only do work. The cost is typically inexpensive compared to living in an assisted living facility. However, if twenty-four-hour care is involved, the pricing will probably rival that of an assisted facility, [12] but at least you will be in your own home. This type of in home living arrangement is excellent and successful as long as you don't have serious cognitive impairment.

Please be aware that there is great demand on all of our senior support services and all nonprofits. They are primarily staffed by unpaid volunteers who are trying to fill the needs of seniors and caregivers. Many social services have told me that often obviously financially capable clients donate very little, saying they want to save all they have to give to their children. Yet the nonprofits that are giving the elders services that their children can't or won't provide are struggling to pay the bills. Look at it this way: The best way for a senior to help their children is to be financially generous in supporting these services that help.

These organizations rise to the need of seniors to enjoy independence while giving their families and friends freedom too. If you can be financially generous to these organizations, please do. You might call it "paying it forward." Your adult children are following behind you, so if these organizations are not financially supported, their services won't be available in the future when your children need them.

In-Home Services

For some, the possibility of hiring in-home help is an option. Finding qualified, reliable services is your goal. If you are considering home healthcare, keep your physician involved. Health insurance plans that cover home-based care (including Medicare and Medicaid) require a physician's orders before they will pay for covered services. The home-care agency can perform important functions for you, such as verifying credentials, checking references, conducting a background check and drug test, and arranging for a substitute or replacement so that your care is not interrupted. This is very important! Interrupted care means the primary caregiver has to be there on a moment's notice to fill in the gaps. Remember, independence for you and *your* family is the goal.

Sources for finding home care providers are: Family Caregiver Alliance (www.caregiver.org) hospital discharge planners, and www.eldercare.gov. Once you have the names of qualified agencies, you may want to check how they compare to other home care providers in your state by logging onto www.medicare.gov. Introduced in November 2003, this website reports on Medicare-certified agencies and how well they accomplish tasks such as helping patients improve dressing, bathing, or walking skills. The reports do not cover all aspects of home care services but can be used in conjunction with other sources of information about the agency. In the worksheet on the following page there is a list of questions that AARP recommends you ask the home health agency, such as, "What accreditations does the agency have?"

Formal In-Home Support Questionnaire

QUESTION	COMMENTS
1. What are the agency's accreditations?*	
2. What is the agency's hiring standards (e.g. background checks, drug tests, etc.)?	
3. How does the agency monitor the quality of care they provide?	
4. What fees will you be charged?	
5. Are additional fees charged for extra services?	
6. What are considered extra services?	
7. Are your services covered by Medicare?	
8. Are they approved to bill and accept payments from Medicare?	
9. Do they have a payment plan?	
10. Do they have a sliding scale for clients in need?	
11. Does this agency have a back-up procedure to assure that care is not interrupted?	
12. What are the agency's problem resolution procedures?	

*An agency may be accredited by the Joint Commission for the Accreditation of Health Organization (JCAHO) or by the Community Health Accreditation Program (CHAP). Both have rigorous standards and review processes.

Note: Either your health insurance plan, Medicare, Medicaid, or the VA may cover some of the basic skilled or unskilled health services. However, you must pay for any services that are not covered or that you arrange on your own.

Medicare

Home-based healthcare services covered by Medicare include: skilled nursing care (nurses or rehabilitation staff who manage, observe, and evaluate your care), various therapies (speech/language, occupational, physical), and part of the cost for renting medical equipment such as wheelchairs, walkers, or oxygen equipment. Personal care—such as help with bathing, management, and cooking—are not usually covered. This care by Medicare is only for one hundred days. After that you will have to pay out of pocket for everything your supplemental insurance does not cover. To find out about Medicare's guidelines for covering home health services, call Medicare toll-free at 1–800–633–4227. Or go to Medicare's website: www.medicare.gov.

Medicaid/Medi-Cal

Medicaid is called Medi-Cal in California. Medicaid covers at-home health services for those who meet certain income and asset guidelines, basically less than $2,000 in assets. Some of the services that may be covered are: outpatient hospital services (therapies administered at home are considered outpatient services), skilled nursing care, and transportation. Some states allow for payment to family members who are caring for their loved one at home. For information about Medicaid coverage in your state, call the Medicaid office in your state.

Veterans

Veterans who have had at least ninety days of wartime duty qualify for temporary financial assistance when they are ill under the Veterans Administration's "Soldiers, Sailors, and Marines Fund." Covered services may include medical supplies, homemaker services, a home health aide, or respite care for family members who care for veterans at home. If the veteran was 100 percent disabled due to service or served twenty or more years of active duty, the veteran's spouse may be eligible for healthcare benefits too.

A popular VA program—VA Aid and Attendance—is for vets who have one day of their ninety days active duty during wartime, less than $90,000 in liquid assets, and are disabled. They or their spouse may be eligible for this benefit. This can amount to as much as $1,800, which is significant for paying for in-home support or supplement income of an assisted living community. The qualifying is done by the VA at no charge. Actually, it is illegal to charge for the qualifying process. (As a consumer caveat, this program has been used as a marketing tool by some insurance companies and financial planners who sell insurance products.) All the information for this program can be found at www.VeteransAdministration.gov as well as the location and phone numbers of local regional VA representatives. Also, every VFW has a service officer who is qualified to help with the paperwork and the qualifying process.

Community-Based Concierge Services

There are a few new community-based concierge services starting across the nation. They are all-encompassing concierge services created by residents of a community who want to grow old in the homes they have lived in for years. Now they can do that with confidence that even as they age they can deal with almost any contingency—large or small—without relying on relatives or friends. These communities create a non-profit organization that helps the members find virtually any service they need from twenty-four-hour nursing care to help with a wayward cat, often at a discounted fee. Beacon Hill has been the frontrunner in this new way of living, and they are very helpful to the other communities starting across the United States. Learn more at www.beaconhillvillage.org.

NOTES

_____

_____

_____

_____

_____

_____

_____

_____

_____

_____

_____

_____

_____

_____

_____

_____

_____

_____

_____

_____

_____

_____

_____

HOME-SAFETY CHECKLIST

The National Institute on Aging (NIA) indicates that falls are the number-one reason for hospitalization, and they seldom "just happen."[13] The NIA says the more you take responsibility for your overall health and well-being, the less likely you are to fall. One-half to two-thirds of all falls occur in or around the home. [14] Find ways to minimize falls around the home if you want to maximize your chances of aging in place. According to the National Center for Injury Prevention and Control, there are four primary things you can do to prevent falls: [15]

1.   Begin a regular exercise program.

2.   Make your home safer.

3.   Have your health care provider review your medicines.

4.   Have your vision checked.

Exercise is the *number-one* factor in achieving good health. If you are not a self-starter when it comes to making yourself exercise, call your local YMCA, senior center, arthritis foundation, or community hospital for suggestions on exercise programs in your area. Making your home safer is an important preemptive step that you need to take. The following are practical solutions to avoiding falls, as suggested by Alan McMillan, the National Safety Council president.

Follow these tips to prevent slips and falls in your home:

1. Keep the floor clear. Reduce clutter, and safely tuck telephone and electrical cords out of walkways.

2. Keep the floor clean. Clean up grease, water, and other liquids immediately. Don't wax floors.

3. Install handrails in stairways. Have grab bars in the bathroom (by toilets and in tub/shower).

4. Make sure living areas are well lit. We can all trip and fall in the dark.

5. Be aware that climbing and reaching high places will increase your chances of a fall. Use a sturdy step stool with handrails when these tasks are necessary.

6. Follow medication dosages closely. Using medication incorrectly may lead to dizziness, weakness, and other side effects. These can all lead to a dangerous fall.

There is no way to anticipate all possibilities for your future needs, but many changes to the home can be anticipated. Almost any aging disability carries with it the potential need for wheelchairs, wheelchair access, bathing safety, functional safe rooms without clutter, and easy main floor access for all daily needs. Acceptance of these probabilities before infirmity will give you greater flexibility in planning your home design. A preplanned design of the home for accessibility and functionality in later life is a necessity to decrease falls and increase the possibility of aging in place. You can make an informal checklist, which you can implement yourself or hire a professional to do for you.

Some states and local areas have education and/or home modification programs to help older people prevent falls.

Check with your local government's health department or division of elder affairs to see if there is a program in your area.

For more complete information on simple, inexpensive repairs and changes that would make your home safer, contact the U.S. Consumer Product Safety Commission at the address below. Ask for a free copy of the booklet *Home Safety Checklist for Older Consumers.* Consumer Product Safety Commission Washington, DC 20207 800–638–2772/800–638–8270 (TTY).

Home Modification/ Universal Design

Now that we have reviewed the basic safety tips, let's go on to discuss more complete safety measures. If you think about it, when you purchased your home you bought it maybe thirty to forty years ago. At that time you were thirty to forty years younger, probably newlyweds or had two or three children. You chose your home based on the comfort and convenience level for that state in your life. Over the years you have probably changed a little; however, you may not have changed your home to meet your current convenience and comfort needs. Remember as I stated in the beginning, a sudden fall often sends individuals to rehab, and they can't go home, because their home will not accommodate a wheelchair-bound individual. *Home modification has become the best solution for aging in place.* The traditional home you were so proud of for its convenience and comfort for the young family won't always take care of you when you break a leg or hurt your back. People need to realize that they need their home to grow old with them. The eighty-two-year-old grandmother is still proud of her home. She just needs to modify it for the comfort and convenience of an eighty-two-year old, not a thirty-year-old mother of three.

The most common problem I have found with recommending home modification is the reluctance of the client to use it, because they have not fully reached the point of accepting their current needs. Many have already compensated their environment in other ways—possibly in unsafe ways—and they don't want to change. Are you using the toilet paper holder to help lift yourself from the commode? Are you not bathing regularly because going upstairs is too difficult? Do you hate to use the dishwasher because it is so low?

If any of these situations sound familiar, it is time for your home to fit your current needs rather than the needs of a young family. After all, it is *your* home! Many people are reluctant to make home modifications because they believe their home will look like an institution. Over the years you may have remodeled, but the contractor didn't mention the alternative of wider doorways or a downstairs full bath, etc. The National Resource Center on Supportive Housing and Home Modification at USC (www.homemods.org) has found, through surveys with individuals, that unless the clients asked for a modification, the contractor didn't offer one. So as pioneers in the age wave, it is up to you to ask. An entire industry of trained home modification experts, contractors, and designers is emerging. In 1977, Michael Bednar coined the phrase "universal design." He noted that the functional capability of all individuals is enhanced when environmental barriers are removed. [16]

Often a reluctance to modify the home is due to the cost of the modifications. One must weigh the cost of living in an assisted or skilled facility to that of actually paying for the changes to be made to their home. As we stated before, acceptance that your physical needs will change is integral to making preparations before the situation is out of your control. If you would really like to live in your home, I would strongly suggest you try to overcome these stumbling blocks. There are a few states that have Medicare waivers that will pay for some modifications. You would have to check with your state Medicare office to find out if that is available.

Some cities have home modification programs available to upgrade some of the seniors' homes, yet they are not very extensive. I recommend you check with your local Medicare office and your local Human Services offices to see if these wonderful programs are available to you prior to seeking the changes on your own.

Here are some of the more common Universal Design features Bednar suggested:

- No-step entry: No one needs to use stairs to get into a universal design home or into the home's main rooms.

- One-story living: Places to eat, use the bathroom, and sleep are all located on one level, which is barrier free.

- Wide doorways: Doorways that are thirty-two to thirty-six inches wide let wheelchairs pass through. They also make it easy to move big things in and out of the house.

- Wide hallways: Hallways should be thirty-six to forty-two inches wide. That way, everyone and everything moves easily from room to room.

- Extra floor space: Everyone feels less cramped, and people in wheelchairs have more space to turn.

Bednar's universal design concept has become increasingly popular for two reasons: First, it looks nice. People with disabilities don't feel like they are settling for an ugly house.

Secondly, people who *don't* have disabilities think that universal homes look and work much better than the old models.

As this is a growing concept, it is important that you make sure you have a knowledgeable home modification expert who knows what is available as well as the proper height, distances, etc., to install assistive devices. Should you need to find advice on what would be best for you, many local physical and or occupational therapists at your local hospital would be a good source for advice. Call and ask if they would mind coming to your home just to give you suggestions. Remember, planning ahead is the key.

The changes you can make to your home are endless: kitchen cabinets with pull-down shelves, closets with adjustable shelves, counters a wheelchair can roll under, good lighting, lever door handles, rocker light switches, etc. You might have a bedroom and bath downstairs but would need a ramp to make your home accessible. Review the possibilities of where a ramp could be quickly installed. Installing the ramp prior to any hospitalization is not necessary, but knowing one can be put in place quickly and who will install it is important.

I've seen remodels that can include decorative bridges in the landscape instead of ramps. All I'm suggesting is take care of the big things now, such as the downstairs bedroom and bathroom. Keep your contractor numbers handy to get the finishing touches quickly if you should need them. If you're looking for a new home or a second home close to the children, you can see the advantage of using these universal design features when you make a list of things you *must have*.

Currently I'm aware of three organizations that certify home modification specialists and advise on universal design. If you want to find someone in your area, try these websites:

1. The National Resource Center on Supportive Housing and Home Modification at USC www.homemods.org.

2. National Home Builders: www.nahb.org/default.aspxand

3. Easy Living: www.easylivinghome.org

On the AARP site www.aarp.org under resources you will find a consumer checklist for long-term independence. You can go through your home and check for adaptations you might need.

When choosing a contractor, be sure to ask for details of past work and recommendations from previous clients. Then obtain and compare quotes from at least three different contractors.

Other Safety Features

You have to be able to take your meds on time to be healthy. There are numerous pillboxes designed to help you. There are a variety of pill dispensers and reminders. The Multi-Alarm Pill Boxes organize all your daily pills and remind you with a loud alarm up to thirty-seven times per day. All pillboxes need to be filled at least once a week; so if you cannot see your medications, you need to add this job to your list of help needed from your support system.

Typically your local human services department can direct you to the local supplier in your area. Taking medication on time is of extreme importance. One of the first changes we see in individuals when they move to assisted living is improved health, due to taking their medications as prescribed.

My mother and my aunt have macular degeneration. They both said they really missed being able to read their watches; we purchased a myriad of watches with various faces, hoping to find the right one. At last we found a watch at Radio Shack that had an alarm every half hour. They both said that was a comfort. Those of us who can see just take for granted those little pleasures.

There is another safety measure available for free in most communities. This measure goes by various names, one of which is "Vial of Life." This is a common pharmacy pill bottle. Within the bottle is a list of all the information a paramedic or fireman might need to help you quickly, if necessary. The list states your medications, your doctor's name, your advance directive, and your primary support person's phone number. This bottle is usually accessible in any community through the local fire department. They may have another name for the service, but they all work the same way. The only difference is that some say put the bottle in the refrigerator and others say put it in the medicine cabinet. However, when they give you the bottle, they will tell you where to keep it for quick access by a medical response team.

I consider *medical alert jewelry* a must when living alone. Usually, you wear a button on a chain around your neck or a wrist bracelet. If you fall or need emergency help, you just push the button to alert the service. If you don't respond when they call, they will call the individual you have listed for emergencies. If that individual doesn't answer his/her call, the emergency staff will be sent to your home.

Many seniors think this device makes them appear old. I actually recommend it for anyone living alone, especially young women. You can't imagine how many seniors I know who tell me stories of having fallen, and they laid on the floor for hours or days because no one could hear them call. There is nothing quite as nice for the price!

Call human services or senior centers first. They will know the least expensive, most effective local systems. Most medical insurance companies and Medicare do not cover items like medical alarm services, so be sure to ask about cost. You will probably have to pay for them yourself. However, even if they cost more, these items can give you more independence. They can also give your caregiver a sense of security that you have everything you need.

There are so many new aids now and more being developed every day. You might want to consider looking at some of the newly developed "assistive devices." You will have more than you can possibly consider.

Hoarding

On the issue of safety often comes the question of hoarding. Hoarding is the excessive collection of items, along with the inability to discard them. Hoarding creates cramped, unsafe living conditions that may fill the home to capacity with only narrow pathways winding through the stacks of clutter.

Hoarders have the inability to discard items. They keep stacks of newspapers, magazines, or junk mail. Papers may be on the stove or in the oven. Vermin can rule in the refuse. This creates a fire and health hazard to the occupant of the home as well as the neighbors. This clutter can be so out of control that local authorities will order the home cleared of the clutter.

Once again, if you want to stay independent and in control of your environment, look around. Do you have only a pathway to your chair and bedroom? Have your family members been commenting on the clutter? Please talk with a doctor. Remember, you want to be in control of your stuff. An excellent resource to find a professional to help de-clutter the home would be the National Association of Senior Move Managers. They have professionals who can work with you and reorganize the clutter. You can reach a professional at www.NASMM.org.

Home Safety
Worksheet A

A. GENERAL QUESTIONS	YES		NO		CHANGES TO BE MADE
1. When climbing and reaching high places, do you use a sturdy step stool with handrails?	Y		N		
2. Do any of your medications cause you dizziness.	Y		N		
3. Are your stairways, hallways and pathways well lighted with easy to reach switches?	Y		N		
4. Are your pathways tidy?	Y		N		
5. Are all carpets fixed firmly to floors?	Y		N		
6. Are there non-slip strips on tile and wooden floors?	Y		N		
7. Are all electric cords and telephone wires near walls and away from walking paths?	Y		N		
8. Are all of your furniture (especially low coffee tables) and other objects placed so they are not in your way when you walk?	Y		N		
9. Are all of your sofas and chairs a good height for you, so that you can get into and out of them easily?	Y		N		

Home Safety Worksheet B

B. BEDROOM QUESTIONS	YES	NO	CHANGES TO BE MADE
1.Have you placed night-lights and light switches close to your bed?	Y	N	
2. Can you reach the telephone from bed?	Y	N	

C. BATHROOM QUESTIONS	YES	NO	CHANGES TO BE MADE
1.Is the bathroom door at least 32" wide?	Y	N	
2.Is someone able to unlock the door from the outside?	Y	N	
3.Does the door open out?	Y	N	
4.Does the bathroom have enough clear floor space for a wheelchair?	Y	N	
5.Does the floor have a non-slip surface?	Y	N	
6.Do you have a telephone in the bathroom that you can reach from the toilet and tub?	Y	N	
7.Is the sink 34 in. from the floor?	Y	N	
8.Does your sink have knee space underneath?	Y	N	
9.Can you control hot and cold water with one handle?	Y	N	

10. Does the sink and shower have an anti-scald device?	Y	N	
11. Is there plenty of counter space to hold all of your things?	Y	N	
12. Is the counter top rounded on the edges?	Y	N	
13. Can you reach your medicine while being seated?	Y	N	
14. Do you have a mirror that tilts up and down?	Y	N	
15. Is the toilet 17 inches from the floor?	Y	N	
16. Does your toilet have grab bars around it?	Y	N	
17. Is there at least 18 inches of free space in front of the toilet?	Y	N	
18. Are there 42 inches of floor space on the side of the toilet?	Y	N	
19. Are you able to reach your toilet paper easily?	Y	N	
20. Does your toilet have a bidet seat, to make cleaning easier?	**Y**	**N**	

NOTES

_____

_____

_____

_____

_____

_____

_____

_____

_____

_____

_____

_____

_____

_____

_____

_____

_____

_____

_____

_____

_____

_____

FINANCIAL
CONSIDERATIONS

Financial planning, living wills, and long-term care insurance will not be covered in depth in this chapter. I will only suggest you use experts in the field of elder law estate planning, financial planning, and tax planning that are *fee for service* individuals. *Fee for service* means they charge you a set price for their services; they are not paid by other companies on commission to sell their products. The old saying, "You get what you pay for," applies here. A financial planner who has a financial stake in the course of action that he/she recommends to a client faces an inherent conflict of interest and cannot be considered objective or unbiased. This is true even if the planner truly believes that he/she has only the best interests of the client at heart.

Unfortunately, the vast majority of financial advisors in the United States are sellers of financial products. Some or all of their income may be dependent upon their ability to steer their clients to a limited number of the thousands of financial products available today. (Putting aside the conflict-of-interest factor, this limiting of choices in and of itself often is enough to impact the quality of the investment advice.)

These advisors include stockbrokers, analysts, insurance agents, accountants, and attorneys, as well as financial planners. Many of their clients are not aware of their advisor's dependence on selling products or do not recognize its significance. NAPFA, the National Association of Personal Financial Advisors believes that many of the problems that beset Americans today in their financial affairs—including the mismanagement of debt, failure to protect retirement assets, and poor allocation of savings and investments—relate directly to the conflicts of interest that pervade the marketplace. Individuals of this association can be found at www.napfa.org.

I mention this because most individuals want to be sure their assets last as long as they do. One of the jobs the elder-law attorney has is to know the rules of government-run programs that may help you. The elder-law attorney will know the asset tests to determine how best to advise and set up your estate. Their task is to stretch your money to last a lifetime. In some cases they cannot do the best for your estate because you have been sold products that will eliminate that option. In my practice, I recommend only a *fee for service* elder-law attorneys. You can find these individuals by going to www.lcplfa.org *and search for the one nearest you. I have experienced the best result from a fee for service financial planner who interfaces with the elder-law attorney to be sure the safest mode of protecting assets is in the client's best interest.*

As for long-term care insurance, most of the seniors I work with are in their eighties plus. It is typically too expensive to start then. If you are in your fifties, it might make sense. Discuss this with your elder-law attorney; they will have the best advice for your situation.

It is currently a well-known demographic in marketing circles that the elderly are not poor, but they are not rich either; more precisely, they are rich in one way and not in another. Typically, their incomes are only half as large as those of younger households, but they have twice the wealth. Most of the elderly are retired, so their incomes consist largely of pensions, Social Security, interest, and dividends. Along with that, they usually have stocks, mutual funds, and savings accounts; and, thanks to appreciation, home equity has been one of the best savings accounts for seniors.

If you want to make adaptations to your home or pay for in-home help, you know that it will take money; or you may be one of the seniors who have to decide between the grocery store and the pharmacy. Either way, you need cash. Now there is a way to convert the equity in your home to cash so that you can continue living in your home for the rest of your life. This financial arrangement is called a reverse mortgage. There are high front-end fees on reverse mortgages that should be considered before taking one, and this has to be balanced against the other factors in your estate to determine a way to make your money last. If you participate in a means-tested program, such as Medicaid or Supplemental Security Income (SSI), choose a payout option from a reverse mortgage loan that delivers payments in fixed monthly amounts versus one lump sum to avoid impacting your eligibility for Medicaid and SSI programs. Once again, it is important to have a professional like an elder-law attorney coordinating the financial as well as legal aspects of making your money last.

As covered in chapter two, you may be eligible for VA aid and attendance, which will help offset some of your income needs.

Doing this preplanning one segment at a time is very difficult. An elder-law attorney specializes in this area and knows the best team to pull together to be sure all the necessary criteria are met.

Fraud

I will never forget one of my first cases I worked on involved a fraud situation in which the client lost her home to investment fraud. She didn't want to share her financial status with her children, but she did share with a salesman at the door. Senior services across the country have indicated to me that this is a big problem.

A California Department of Corporations study found that 70 percent of Californians over the age of fifty have been approached by a fraudulent individual. The study found seniors seem to be the most vulnerable to fraud for several reasons: 1) seniors tend to be home more often and isolated from family and friends; 2) seniors tend to be more trusting and more easily intimidated, less apt to be rude; and 3) seniors tend to have a substantial amount of disposable income. (Remember, these income demographics are well known.) Please, please, if you don't want to share your information with your children, follow the advice of (SAIF), seniors against investment fraud. This is an innovative educational outreach program led by the Department of Corporations available in California. SAIF says, "A knowledgeable consumer is a 'safe' consumer."

They say don't invest until you have completed the "Four C's":

- Call SAIF first: 1–866–275–2677
- Consider all your options
- Compare the product to others
- Consult with someone you trust

SAIF offers a few basic self-defense tips:

1. Don't be a "courtesy victim." Con artists don't hesitate to take advantage of people with good manners who fear they are being rude by hanging up or saying no to their sales pitches. (I personally have one standing rule. If someone is selling at the door or on the phone, the answer is no. Any sales person who cannot wait a minimum of twenty-four hours for you to check him out—the answer is no.)

2. Be wary of unsuspected phone calls, letters, or personal visits from strangers who require your immediate investment. Turn down any high-pressure requests that are accompanied by immediate action warnings like, "Tomorrow will be too late," or "You must act now." If the person offering you an investment opportunity is not willing to give you time to investigate the salesperson or the firm and investment opportunity itself, then there is probably something that they are trying to hide from you. Call SAIF for advice. Remember, legitimate financial counselors are proud of their license and reputation; they don't mind you checking.

3. Always ask for written information about the organization behind the investment plan. This includes the work history and background of the person handling your account as well as information on the firm itself. Make sure your brokers, investment advisers, and investment advisor representatives are licensed to sell securities. Don't be afraid to ask questions. If the salesperson does not want to give you information, it is because they are hiding something.

Lastly, SAIF says don't let embarrassment or fear keep you from reporting investment fraud or abuse or from asking questions about your investment. Con artists prey on your fears and rely on them in order to con you out of your financial freedom. They are counting on your fear to make their money. If you feel any doubt about an investment or feel that you have been a victim of investment fraud, report such fears immediately. These con artists will stop at nothing until they take everything you have.

SAIF is a California non-profit organization to serve the California seniors. However, if you can't find your state's program, call your local area Council on Aging for direction or call your state's Department of Corporations.

Summary

Please note that a fall in your home would be the most likely cata-lyst to take you from your home surroundings to an institutional setting. I have repeatedly suggested this is the number-one cause of hospitalization for seniors, because it is my hope you will take time to look at your home and prepare for any potential hazards. Almost everyone is happier in his/her own space and with the indepen-dence that goes with it.

The concept of all of these pre-planning techniques is intended to insure your independence and ability to stay in your home. Whether you are preparing your home for safety, looking for financial support, or legal support, the answers are here. Your local Area Council on Aging is also one of the best phone calls you can make to find your local resources. They are non-profit and have only your best interest at heart. Remember, if you wait until an incident happens, you will have planned for disaster. It would be unwise to make the assumption you will be the one in only a few who doesn't have mobility or sight impairments in late life. You as well as your caregivers will be overwhelmed. You will have made the choice to minimize your chances of staying in your home and thus give up the independence you so desire.

I hope this book is a joy and an excellent starting point for you to "age in place" wherever you choose. I wish you only a safe, long, and happy life in your home.

NOTES

ABOUT THE AUTHOR

Donna Christner-Lile is a San Francisco Bay area life transitions consultant. Her counseling practice, Christner-Lile Consulting^SM, is more than a business; it is a mission as well as a tribute to God for her good health and happiness gleaned from her experience traversing mid-life. She says part of the secret to handling transitions well is allowing yourself to do something you *want* to do, over and above what you *have* to do.

Donna knew how to balance life, career, and education. That seemed like enough; however, life changes, and unexpectedly she became a caregiver to her ninety-two-year-old mother. She was able to experience firsthand what many sandwich generation individuals go through. She knows from experience that unexpected changes are often the very best. Her time with her mother was a nurturing experience for mother and daughter—a time they both will always cherish. There would have been a great loss for both of them had they not had time to come together in late life.

With increasing numbers of boomers facing caregiver stress, downsizing, and retirement issues, as well as elders choosing to remain in their homes, the need for a counselor like Donna, who can coordinate the resources to help, is great.

She has successfully combined her experience and education gleaned from two life careers into the best planning resource for boomers, caregivers, and elders. She was the executive director of a nonprofit organization, Counseling Life Transitions. Through that organization she helped seniors identify and implement assistive technologies and services in their home for safety and comfort or suggested they find a safer environment in which to live.

Donna has a bachelor's degree in Lifespan Human Development and a master's in Life Transitions Counseling. She is a national certified counselor (NCC) and a member of the American Counseling Association.

END NOTES

1   Susan Martin, Ph.D., "Tweens and Teens: Generations United,"
    Harris Interactive (July, 2005): www.harrisinteractive.com/news/
    newsletters/k12news/HI_Trends&Tudes News2005_v4_iss07.pdf

2   Karen Goldberg Goff, "Relatively Close" *The*
    Washington Times (Aug, 15, 2004).

3   http://www.nsc.org/injuryfacts/preview.pdf National Safety
    Council Injury Facts,
    (2005–2006 Edition)

4   National Safety Council Analysis of National Center for Injury
    Prevention and Control Injury Surveillance Data Using WIS-
    CARS™ (2006) (http:/www.CDC.GOV/NCIPC/WISCARS/)

5   Sharon Tennstedt, "Family Caregiing in an
    Aging Society" paper presented at U.S.Administration on
    Aging Symposium: Longevity in the New Century. Bal-
    timore, MD. (March, 29, 1999) http://www.aoa.gov

6   Source:Peter S.Arno, "Economic Value of Informal Care-
    giving: 2000," presented at the American Association
    of Geriatric Psychiatry, Orlando, Florida. (February 24,
    2002) http://www.nfcacares.org/pdfs/pa2000.ppt

7   John Weicher, "Life in a Gray America,
    "Outlook (Fall 1998) issues.

8   Suzanne Martin, Ph.D., Source: Harris Interactive
     Youth Query[sm] May 18–23, 2005, *Trends and Tudes* (July
     2005) http://www.harrisinteractive.com/news/newslet-
     ters/k12news/HI Trends&TudesNews2005 v4 iss07.pdf

9   Suzanne Martin, Ph.D., Source: Harris Interactive Youth
     Query[sm] May 18–23, 2005, *Trends and Tudes* (July 2005) http://
     retention.harrisblackintl.com/news/newsletters/k12news/
     HI_Trends&TudesNews2005_v4_iss07.pdf. Editorial: Our
     Take On it, Suzanne Martin, PH.D. Harris Interactive

10   Metropolitan Life Insurance Company, "Balancing Caregiving
     with Work and the Cost involved," Findings from a National
     Study by the National Alliance for Caregiving and the National
     Center on Women and Aging at Brandeis University. (November
     1999) http://www.metlife.com/WPSAssets/12949500261100547

11   Dale Atkins, *I'm OK, You're My Parents: How to Overcome Guilt,
     Let Go of Anger, and Create
     a Relationship That Works* (New York: Henry
     Holdan Company, LLC 2004)

12   "Preventing Falls and Fractures" National *Institute on Aging Age
     Page* (June 2004) http://www.
     niapublications.org/agepages/falls.asp

13   M.C. Nevitt, S.R. Cummings, S. Kidd, D. Black. "Risk Factors for
     Recurrent Nonsyncopal Falls. A prospective study." *Journal of the
     American
     Medical Association.*

14   Centers for Disease Control and Prevention. "Falls
     Among Older Adults: summary of research find-
     ings." (January, 2005) http://www.cdc.gov

15   The National Center for Injury Preven-
     tion and Control http://www.cdc.gov/injury

16   Michael Bednar, "Barrier Free Environments,"
     Stroudsburg, Pa.: Dowden, Hutchison, and Ross (1977)
     http://www.arch.virginia.edu/faculty/MichaelJBednar

NOTES

_____
_____
_____
_____
_____
_____
_____
_____
_____
_____
_____
_____
_____
_____
_____
_____
_____
_____
_____
_____
_____
_____
_____
_____

_____

_____

_____

_____

_____

_____

_____

_____

_____

_____

_____

_____

_____

_____

_____

_____

_____

_____

_____

_____

_____

_____

_____

_____

_____

CPSIA information can be obtained at www.ICGtesting.com
Printed in the USA
BVOW07s0917041213

338068BV00009B/317/P